2020 YEAR OF THE NURSE

A Nurse's Journey
through the Frontlines

Martha Hoy

Based on True events.

ISBN | 9781736267042

CONTENTS

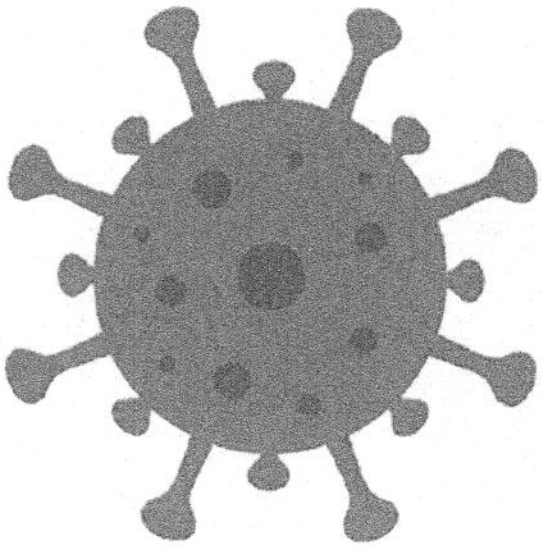

Dedicated to all nurses and frontline workers who persevered through 2020.

In memory of my friend Penny Anderson—a nurse, EMT/ Paramedic, and humanitarian who helped shape my career. To my Chicago family for supporting me through 2025 when I had just one good arm, so I could finish this book: Richard Costello, an angel sent from God.

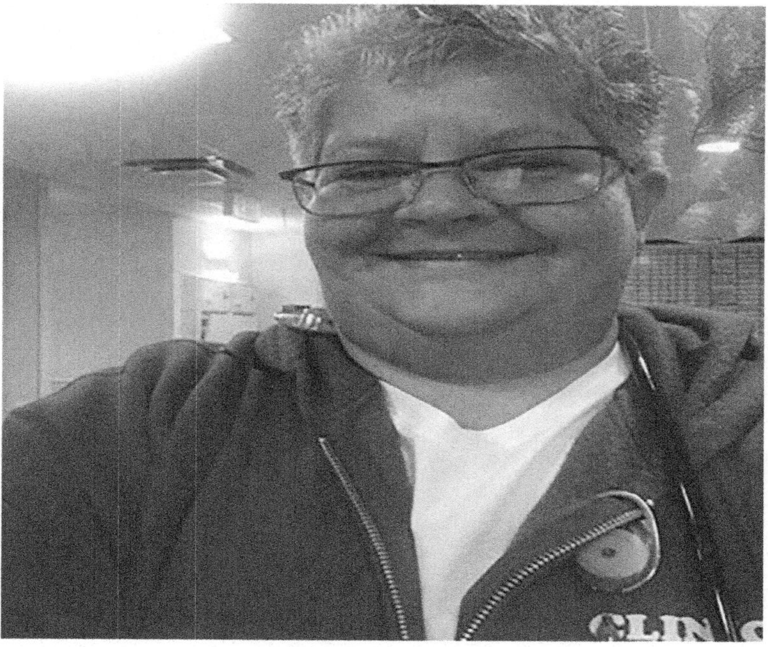

INTRODUCTION

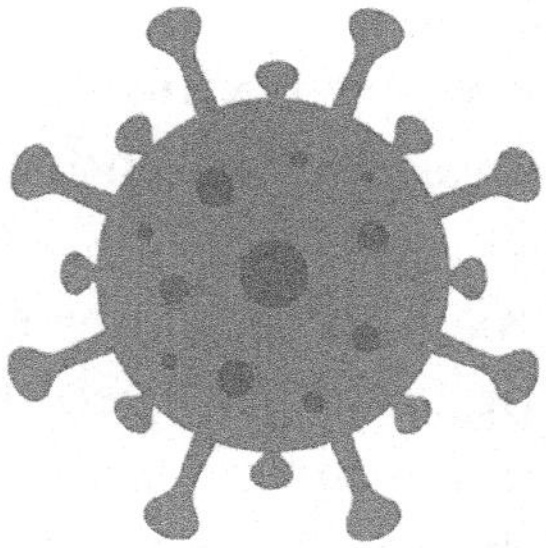

My aspiration to become a nurse began in childhood, inspired by caring for my bed-bound grandfather. Reading to him and spending time together fostered my love for reading, writing, and nursing. Growing up in a small West Virginia town, I watched my grandfather, Edward "Ted," work hard as a coal miner and farmer, leaving school in third grade to support his family. Those early experiences shaped my calling.

During the pandemic, I served on the frontlines in Las Vegas, Nevada. In my memoir "Becoming Mother Martha," I recount how Vegas became my refuge after fleeing danger in 2018, and how it offered me a chance to serve others. I am proud of my profession and of how nurses and healthcare workers responded to the 2020 crisis. This book aims to share the experience of being a nurse during such a tumultuous time. I focus solely on lived experiences—without opinions or speculations about the pandemic's origins. Questions about COVID-19 may remain unanswered for decades.

Regardless of one's perspective, Covid-19 affected everyone. Illness, loss of work, financial hardship, grief, and quarantine touched lives worldwide. News broadcasts served as constant reminders of the crisis beyond our walls.

My goal is to give nurses a voice by sharing what 2020 looked like from inside the hospital. I hope to spark conversation and perhaps inspire change in healthcare. What nurses learned quickly became textbook knowledge, but I want future healthcare professionals to understand the human experience.

As a child, I never imagined a global pandemic or that I would fight to keep people alive. This book is a generalization of what most nurses experienced to protect the privacy of others yet show the reality faced by nurses, doctors, and healthcare professionals in 2020.

I hope you enjoy this story. I sure did enjoy the journey.

Much love,
Martha Hoy, RN

CHAPTER ONE

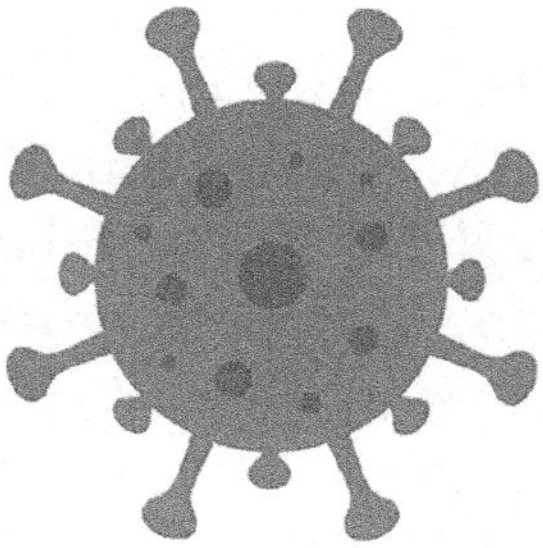

Before the Storm

"It was the best of times; it was the worst of times." – Charles Dickens

Before March 2020, the hospital felt predictable.

Not easy—never easy—but familiar in the way that long routines become a second heartbeat. You learned the rhythm of the unit, the rise and fall of call lights, the steady beeping of monitors that blended into background noise. You knew which rooms were always colder than the rest, which IV pumps were temperamental. Where to stand so you could catch the morning sun through the nurses' station windows. There was comfort in that kind of knowing.

Shift change was orderly in those days. Reports were given with coffee in hand, pens clicking, charts flipped open in practiced rhythm. We talked about patient labs, wound care, discharges, and admissions. We complained about being short-staffed even then, about charting systems that froze at the worst times, about insurance refusing coverage for patients who clearly needed care. But it was the good kind of complaining—the familiar kind. The kind that meant things were normal.

We still laughed. Loudly, sometimes.

Inside our unit, humor was survival long before the world knew it would need it. We joked at the nurses' station, shared snacks, celebrated birthdays with grocery store cake, and left notes on lockers for coworkers going through hard weeks. There was a rhythm to our days—med passes, assessments, admissions, discharges—and it made sense. It had shape. It had edges.

Then one morning during report, our charge nurse mentioned something new.

"By the way…there's this virus in China," she said, flipping through her clipboard like it was just another line item. "They say it's bad. Respiratory. Just keep an ear out."

China felt far away in those moments. Like something happening on a different planet. We nodded, half-listened, and returned to discussing potassium levels and discharge plans.

A virus from China didn't change how we worked that day.

We still walked from room to room and in the hallways without masks. We still stethoscoped chests without thinking twice. We still sat shoulder to shoulder in the breakroom, scrolling our phones and sipping coffee from shared pots. If there was danger on the horizon, it was too distant to make a sound.

The hospital was still full of families then. Children running down hallways before being redirected by staff. Spouses sleeping in chairs next to beds. Patients complaining about hospital food. Nurses holding hands during difficult conversations with loved ones present. The unit buzzed with life—messy, chaotic, real life.

The idea that one day those hallways would be eerily quiet, stripped of visitors and heavy with grief, seemed impossible. If someone had told us then what was coming—what we would witness, what we would lose, how we would change—we wouldn't have believed them.

Morale was strong in its own imperfect way. We trusted our systems. We trusted our supplies. We trusted that our hospital could handle anything. Pandemics belonged to history books, not our breakroom TV.

Back then, we planned vacations. We talked about summer. We made dinner reservations and bought concert tickets. We complained about traffic and weather and double shifts, but went on living our lives without fear.

It's strange how clearly I can remember that version of the world now—the one where breathing was just breathing and not something to be taken for granted.

We didn't know it then, but we were standing in the quiet right before impact. The last deep breath before the water closed over our heads.

Before the storm.

CHAPTER TWO

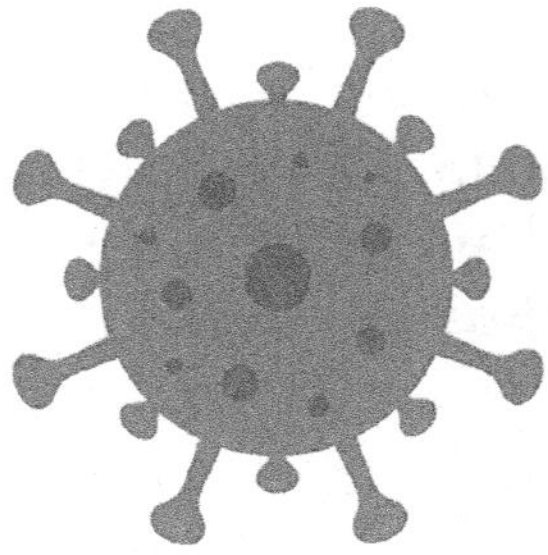

Whispers in the Hallway

"I can feel it coming in the air tonight." – Phil Collins.

In the first weeks of 2020, the hospital hallways took on a strange kind of quiet—not the calm quiet of a slow shift, but the uneasy silence that settles before an approaching storm. It started as a rumor, almost like background noise. A nurse in the break room would mention a headline they saw on their phone. A doctor walking down the hall would murmur something about a new virus overseas. At first, it all felt far away, like a distant weather pattern that might change course before it reached us.

But every day, the whispers grew louder.

Co-workers passed each other at the nurse's station with half-formed questions in our eyes. *Have you heard anything new? Is this real? Should we be worried?* At first, nobody said it out loud. It felt almost wrong to give shape to the fear, as if naming it would make it real. Instead, we smiled tight little smiles, pretending everything was normal, pretending our hands weren't shaking the tiniest bit as we charted or prepped an IV.

Emails began trickling in from administration—short, strangely vague messages about "monitoring developments" and "remaining prepared," words that managed to say a lot without committing to anything. Every update felt like it was written through gritted teeth. They reassured us that the hospital had "protocols in place," though none of us knew what those protocols were. On some shifts, it felt like the only protocol was *don't ask too many questions yet.*

The conversations about PPE were the most frustrating. In January, nobody wanted to talk about masks. Not the higher-ups, not the inventory staff, not even the safety officers. If you asked about stock, you got a carefully rehearsed answer: "We have what we need." If you pressed a little harder, the tone tightened. "Let's not jump ahead." There was this unspoken pressure to stay calm, to not be the one who stirred the pot. But underneath the surface was a quiet, pulling fear: *What if we don't have enough?*

One afternoon, I walked past the supply room and saw two managers huddled inside, their voices low and clipped. I pretended not to listen, but I caught fragments—words like "shortage," "conservation," "if it spreads here." I kept walking, but those words clung to me for the rest of the shift.

By February, it was impossible to ignore. We started seeing new flyers taped to the walls near the elevators—guidelines that seemed to change every other day. Transmission airborne. No, droplets. Masks are required only for suspected cases. No, masks are discouraged for routine care. We'd gather in small groups between patient rooms, trading information the way people trade secrets during wartime. Everyone had heard something different, and the contradictions made the air feel even heavier. We weren't just fighting the unknown—we were fighting confusion.

Nobody wanted to admit it outright, but we could feel something closing in. It was in the way our supervisors avoided eye contact when we asked direct questions. It was in the sudden rationing of N95s—issued only "when appropriate," though no one could tell us what "appropriate" meant. It was in the nervous laugh someone let out when the first staff member said, "Maybe we should get ready."

Mostly, it was in the silence—those long, uneasy pauses after shift huddles, when we looked at each other and felt the weight of what wasn't being said.

Inside our unit, the work was the same. Morning assessments. Medication passes. Charting that never seemed to end. Patients admitted for everything we already knew how to manage—CHF exacerbations, post-surgical recoveries, infections we could name and treat with confidence.

We trusted what we knew.

But slowly, the tone began to change.

Emails started coming more frequently. Infection control updates. New screening questions. Travel history suddenly mattered in a way it never had before.

"Any recent travel outside the country?"

"Any exposure to someone who has traveled?"

We added the questions to our routines, almost mechanically. Most patients answered no. Some didn't know. It didn't seem significant yet—just another box to check, another protocol to follow.

Then came the masks.

At first, it was subtle. A suggestion. Then a recommendation. Then a quiet expectation.

"Wear a mask if the patient has respiratory symptoms."

We weren't alarmed. We had dealt with flu seasons before. We had handled outbreaks. This felt like an extension of something familiar—something we could manage.

But beneath that familiarity, something didn't sit right.

The reports from other places—Italy, New York—began to filter in. Hospitals overwhelmed. Patients flooding ICUs. Words like *shortages* and *ventilators* started appearing more often.

We talked about it in passing.

"Did you see what's happening over there?"

"Yeah, but that's not here."

Not yet.

There was a moment—I don't remember the exact day, just the feeling—when the conversation shifted from curiosity to concern.

It showed up in questions.

"What if this spreads here?"

"Do we even have enough supplies?"

"Are we ready for something like that?"

No one answered directly. Not because they didn't want to—but because no one really knew.

Protocols began to change more frequently.

New guidelines on PPE. Updated isolation procedures. Emails that contradicted the ones sent just days before. It created a quiet uncertainty, the kind that builds slowly, layer by layer.

We started paying closer attention.

Watching the news between tasks. Checking updates on our phones during breaks. Listening more carefully during report, waiting for new information that might change how we worked that day.

And still, patients came and went as they always had.

The rhythm of the unit continued—but it felt slightly off, like a familiar song played just a fraction too slow.

There was more cleaning. More caution. More awareness of coughs, fevers, anything that didn't quite fit.

We began to notice each other more, too.

The way someone lingered after report, asking one more question. The way conversations stretched longer, less about routine and more about uncertainty. The way laughter still happened—but softer, shorter, like it had lost some of its ease.

It wasn't fear yet.

It was anticipation.

The kind that sits just beneath the surface, waiting for something to confirm it.

Then the words started appearing more often.

"Community spread."

"Possible exposure."

"Prepare."

Prepare for what?

That was the question no one could fully answer.

Looking back, those weeks feel suspended in time. We were still standing in the world we understood, but we could see something forming just beyond it—something larger, something we couldn't quite define.

We were watching it approach in real time, piece by piece, without fully grasping what it would become.

If there was a moment when everything could have felt different—when we might have braced ourselves more, prepared more, understood more—it was then.

But hindsight doesn't exist in the moment.

In the moment, we were nurses doing our jobs, adjusting to new information, trusting that whatever came, we would handle it the way we always had.

We didn't know yet that this would be different.

That the rules would keep changing.
That the systems we trusted would be tested.
That the routines we relied on would disappear.

We were still standing in the space between knowing and not knowing.

Between normal and something else.

The early warnings weren't loud.

They didn't need to be.

They were quiet, steady, and persistent—like the first drops of rain before a storm you don't yet realize is coming.

In the hallways, the whispers no longer sounded like rumors. They sounded like warnings. And though the storm hadn't hit yet, we could feel the wind shifting. Something was coming. Something big. Something we weren't prepared for—no matter what the emails said.

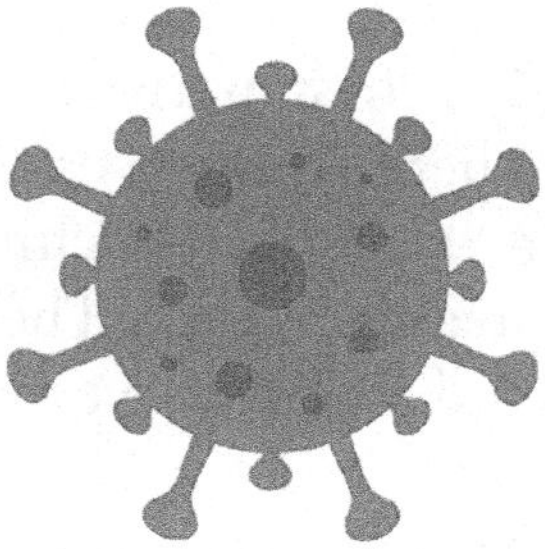

CHAPTER THREE

March 13, 2020—The World Shut Down

“March 2020 the day the Earth stood still.” -WSJ Opinion

It started like any other shift—coffee in hand, report sheets folded into pockets, the low hum of monitors filling the background. But there was something different in the air that morning. You could feel it before anyone said a word. The unit wasn’t as loud. Conversations were shorter. Eyes lingered a little longer than usual.

By the time shift report started, the tension had a name.

“We’ve got our first confirmed COVID patient.”

The words landed heavy. Final.

For weeks, we had heard about it—this virus, distant and abstract, something happening somewhere else. But now it was here. Not on the news. Not across the ocean. Here. In our hospital. On our unit.

Everything after that felt like it moved too fast and not fast enough at the same time.

The first patient arrived differently than any other admission. There was no casual roll-in, no easy chatter. Staff gathered at a distance, watching, adjusting masks that suddenly didn't feel strong enough. The patient struggled to breathe, each inhale sharp and shallow, eyes wide with a fear that didn't need explaining.

Then more came.

By midday, it was clear this wasn't going to be contained to one room, one case, one shift. The admissions stacked up, one after another, like a wave building force. The ER was already filling. Phone calls rang nonstop. Leadership meetings stretched into emergency briefings. Words like *lockdown*, *isolation*, and *pandemic* were no longer theoretical—they were immediate.

Rules began changing in real time.

"No visitors," came one announcement.

"Save your PPE," came another.

"Reuse your masks."

We looked at each other, unsure if we had heard correctly. Reuse? These were items we had been trained to discard after every patient. Now we were being told to fold them carefully, place them in paper bags, and use them again. It went against everything we knew.

But there weren't enough.

That truth settled in quickly and uncomfortably. Supplies that once seemed endless had limits. Masks were counted. Gowns were monitored. Hand sanitizer stations were refilled as fast as they emptied. Every piece of protection became something to guard, to stretch, to make last longer than it was ever meant to.

Fear spread just as fast as the virus.

Not loud, not panicked—but steady, creeping. It showed up in the way nurses hesitated for a split second before entering a room. In the extra time spent adjusting a mask. In the quiet questions:

"Do you think this is enough?"
"What if we bring it home?"
"Are we safe?"

No one had answers.

Outside the hospital, the world was beginning to react. Schools were closing. Businesses were shutting down. Grocery stores were being cleared out. The word *lockdown* started appearing everywhere. Inside the hospital, we didn't have time to process any of it. We were already in it.

And then came the moment that changed everything.

The first COVID death on our unit. Death is something nurses deal with daily, but this was different. This patient came to the hospital with mild symptoms, cough, low-grade fever, and generalized weakness. Just 12 hours later, a Code Blue was called. A sudden change like nothing anyone had ever seen. A large drop in blood pressure and their oxygen saturation. Just like the scenes in the medical dramas on TV, nurses and doctors rushed into the patient's room. Unlike those scenes, the staff was wearing PPE from head to toe: hair caps, N-95 masks, gowns, gloves, and shoe protection. But the urgency was the same, the code blue was the same. Every life-saving measure was performed, but without success. It was just under an hour, but it felt like an eternity. A voice from a corner of the room, from the attending physician could be heard, "Stop all efforts, time of death 18:40."

It happened without ceremony, without the presence of family, without the familiar rituals that usually surrounded the end of a life. Just the sound of machines, the stillness of a room, and a small group of us standing there, trying to absorb what had just happened.

We didn't know what the exact protocol was yet. Even that was unclear. Instructions had changed twice that day already. But what we did know—what we all felt—was that this was only the beginning.

We weren't even fully sure how to handle the body. Protocols were changing so quickly that the instructions we received that morning differed from the ones we received that afternoon. What I remember most is the silence. No family at the bedside. No warm hands holding theirs. Just the beeping of machines slowly going flat-lined and a small team of us standing there, feeling the weight of a life lost without the rituals or gentleness we were used to offering.

No one said it out loud, but it hung in the air between us:

If this is the first... how many more are coming?

Afterward, the unit felt different. Quieter. Heavier. Like something invisible had settled over all of us. Some nurses cried in private. Others kept moving, task to task, as if stopping would make it real in a way they couldn't handle yet.

There was no time to grieve.

There were more patients. More alarms. More uncertainty.

By the end of the shift, exhaustion had already set in—not the kind that comes from physical work, but the kind that comes from carrying something too big to fully understand. Walking out of the hospital that night felt surreal. The world outside didn't match what we had just experienced inside.

The parking lot was still. The sky looked the same. But nothing felt the same.

We sat in our cars in the parking before turning the key, hands resting on the steering wheel, resting and trying to process what had happened during the shift, many times a single thought kept repeating:

This is bigger than us.

March 13, 2020 was the day the line was crossed. The day the unknown became real. The day we stopped preparing and started surviving.

The day the storm arrived.

The day we stopped being ordinary nurses and became witnesses to history. Caregivers in a crisis, no one fully understood. Human beings, trying to stay brave in a world that suddenly felt very fragile.

It still sits on a person's chest like a weight. It was the day everything changed—quietly at first, then all at once. The fear began to build. It was quiet, hidden behind glances exchanged over the tops of surgical masks, behind the way people washed their hands twice, then a third time. We were told to reuse masks that were meant to be disposable. "Conserve PPE," they said. "Make it last." We locked our N95s in paper bags with our names written in black markers, as if ownership could make them safer or cleaner. No one said it aloud, but we all knew: this wasn't enough protection for what we were facing.

Hallway huddles became our new form of communication. A manager would rush out of a meeting with fresh rules—no visitors, new screening protocols, cancel elective surgeries—only for another manager to contradict or revise them twenty minutes later. Nobody was to blame; nobody actually knew what the right thing was. Still, it left us feeling exposed, unprepared, and strangely alone despite being surrounded by coworkers.

The public panic seeped in through every doorway. Phones at the front desk rang relentlessly as families demanded answers we didn't have. The grocery store shelves were already empty of toilet paper and hand sanitizer, and nurses traded stories of driving to five different places before a shift just to find bleach wipes. Some people outside were minimizing the virus; others were convinced the world was ending. Inside the hospital, we existed in a sharp, suspended reality—focused, frightened, and trying to keep each other steady.

We were dealing with the same issues everyone else was dealing with on the outside. Every day, we got dressed to face the very thing the entire world feared. Soldiers in a war in which we knew little about the enemy. An enemy we had no weapons to fight against. While balancing patient care and keeping ourselves safe.

From March 13 into April, it felt like two realities were unfolding at the same time.

Outside the hospital, the world was shutting down. Inside the hospital, everything was opening up in the worst possible way.

The streets grew quiet. Schools were closed. Businesses locked their doors. People stayed home, watching the news, refreshing their phones, trying to understand what was happening.

Inside the hospital, we didn't have the luxury of watching.

We were living it.

Every shift felt like stepping into something that had already accelerated overnight. The patients kept coming—faster than we could process, faster than we could prepare. What had started as a few isolated cases became a steady stream, then a surge.

The same symptoms. The same fear.

"I can't breathe."

It became the phrase we heard over and over again. Different voices, same desperation. It echoed through rooms, through hallways, through our minds long after we left.

We were learning in real time.

There was no handbook for this. No clear protocol that stayed consistent long enough to feel reliable. One day we were told one thing, the next day it changed. PPE guidelines shifted. Isolation rules tightened. Then tightened again.

At some point, we stopped trying to memorize the rules and just adapted as we went.

Masks became constant. Not just for certain patients—for everyone. The first time we wore one for an entire shift, it felt like we were suffocating. By the end of April, it felt like a part of our faces.

We weren't treating COVID so much as we were trying to keep people alive long enough for their bodies to fight it.

There was no clear roadmap.

No standard protocol we trusted. No medication we could point to and say, *this works*. Everything felt experimental, cautious, and often contradictory. What we did one week, we questioned the next.

At the bedside, that uncertainty was its own kind of weight.

Patients came in with the same story—fever, cough, fatigue—and then, suddenly, something would shift. Their oxygen levels would drop quickly, sometimes without warning. You would walk into a room expecting to check vitals, and instead you found someone gasping, their chest rising and falling too fast, eyes wide with fear.

"I can't breathe."

Those words became constant.

Our first line of defense wasn't a medication—it was oxygen. Nasal cannula, then higher flow, then non-rebreather masks. We turned the oxygen up, watched the numbers, adjusted again. Sometimes it worked for a while. Sometimes it didn't.

Proning became routine—turning patients onto their stomachs to help their lungs expand. We coached them through it, repositioning pillows, encouraging them to stay that way as long as they could tolerate.

"Just a little longer," we would say.
"Breathe slow. Stay with me."

Some patients improved with these measures. Many didn't.

And then came the ventilators.

There was a moment—quiet but unmistakable—when you knew a patient was heading in that direction. Their oxygen needs climbed higher and higher. Their breathing became more labored. Conversations shortened to single words, then nods, then just eye contact.

Intubation wasn't just a procedure. It felt like a threshold.

We prepared the room carefully, knowing the risk it carried—not just for the patient, but for us. Fewer people went in. PPE was checked and rechecked. The door closed.

And afterward, the room changed.

The patient lay still, connected to machines that breathed for them. Sedated. Silent. The human connection reduced to numbers on a monitor and the rise and fall of a ventilator.

In those early months, going on a ventilator often felt like a turning point we couldn't reverse.

We didn't have much else to offer.

There were medications being tried—some familiar, some not. Drugs repurposed from other illnesses. Conversations about antivirals, about treatments we hoped might help. But there was no consistency yet. No certainty.

We gave what we could, monitored closely, adjusted constantly.

But most of our care was **supportive**.

Fluids. Oxygen. Positioning. Monitoring. Waiting.

Waiting was the hardest part.

Waiting to see if their oxygen would stabilize.
Waiting to see if their body would respond.
Waiting to see if they would turn a corner—or decline.

As nurses, we are trained to act, to intervene, to fix when something is wrong. But during those months, so much of what we did felt like holding the line—doing everything possible while knowing it might not be enough.

At the bedside, time felt different.

You spent longer in rooms, even when you tried not to. Adjusting oxygen, repositioning, checking again, and watching the monitor for any sign of improvement. Talking to patients through layers of PPE, hoping your voice still felt human behind the mask.

You became very aware of your presence. Especially in the moments when patients asked, "I am going to make it?' after being told they had COVID-19.

Sometimes, your presence was the only comfort you could offer.

There were no families at the bedside. No familiar voices. No hands to hold except ours. And even that was limited—gloved, cautious, brief.

So, we stayed longer when we could.

We talked more.
Explained more.
Reassured, even when we weren't sure ourselves.

Because fear was everywhere—in the patients, in the rooms, in us.

Every shift carried the same quiet question:

Is this the one who will make it?

Some did.

They stabilized. Their oxygen needs decreased. They avoided the ventilator. Those moments felt like small victories—fragile, but real.

But many didn't.

And without clear treatments, without a reliable way to change the outcome, those losses felt heavier. Not because we didn't try—but because we had so few tools to fight with.

Looking back, what stands out most isn't just what we didn't have medically—it's what we had to become in the absence of it.

We became watchers.
Supporters.
Witnesses.

We stood at the bedside in a time when medicine didn't yet have answers, and we gave everything we could anyway.

Not because it was enough.

But because it was all we had.

The isolation was one of the most difficult parts.

Patients were alone in a way that felt unnatural. No family at the bedside. No familiar voices filling the room. Just us—covered in layers of protection, faces hidden, voices muffled.

We tried to fill the gap.

We held phones so families could speak through screens. We repeated messages when connections dropped. We stood in silence while final words were said through an iPad, knowing it wasn't enough, knowing it was all we had.

Outside, new words and phrases were being used —*quarantine, lockdown, social distancing*.

Inside, those words had weight.

Quarantine meant coworkers disappearing from the schedule overnight after an exposure.

Lockdown meant no one coming in, no one going out, a sealed environment where everything stayed contained—including the fear.

Social distancing was impossible. We worked shoulder to shoulder, moving quickly, relying on each other in ways that left no space for distance.

There was fear, but it wasn't loud.

It showed up in quiet questions:

"Did I do that right?"

"Was that enough protection?"

"Am I bringing this home?"

We developed routines outside of work that mirrored the tension inside it. Shoes left at the door. Scrubs removed immediately. Showers taken before touching anything or anyone. A constant awareness that we might carry something invisible with us.

Some nurses isolated from their own families. Slept in separate rooms. Avoided hugs. Lived in a kind of emotional distance that was just as heavy as the physical one.

We were caring for patients while also trying to protect the people we loved from ourselves.

Exhaustion came quickly.

Not just from the work, but from the uncertainty. From the constant vigilance. From the mental load of trying to stay one step ahead of something that kept changing.

Days blurred together. It was hard to remember what happened on which shift, which patient was when. Everything merged into one continuous experience of movement, urgency, and adaptation.

And still, some moments broke through.

A patient stabilizing when you thought they wouldn't. A coworker making you laugh unexpectedly. A brief second of stillness in a supply room where you could close your eyes and just breathe.

Those moments didn't fix anything.

But they kept you grounded.

By April, we understood something we hadn't fully grasped in March:

This wasn't temporary.

This wasn't something that would pass in a few weeks and return us to normal.

This was something else entirely.

Something bigger. Longer. Heavier.

Outside, the world was learning how to stay home.

Inside, we were learning how to endure.

And somewhere between those two realities, we kept showing up—carrying both at the same time, even when it felt like more than we could hold.

CHAPTER FOUR

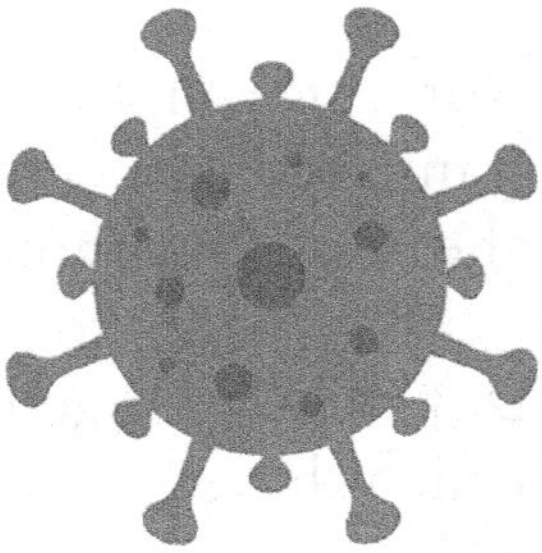

THE INSIDE WAS A WAR ZONE, OUTSIDE THE EARTH STOOD STILL

"You cannot be brave if you have had only wonderful things happen to you." – Mary Tyler Moore.

By April, the hospital no longer felt like a place of healing or the place we always knew. It felt like a war zone—except there were no sirens outside, no smoke in the air, no frontlines you could point to. Just the slow, suffocating crush of patients pouring in with the same desperate look in their eyes: *I can't breathe.*

Most days, we were already over capacity before the morning huddle. The ER was a pipeline of stretchers waiting for beds that didn't exist. Rooms meant for one patient held two, sometimes three. Hallways became makeshift care spaces, with curtains strung up like thin shields between life and death. The sound of oxygen alarms blended into the constant hum of vents, creating a kind of white noise that wrapped itself around your nerves until you couldn't tell if the buzzing was the machines or your own brain misfiring.

Patients were given numbers on arrival at the ER. On the overhead intercom, there were announcements of the number followed by the words either positive or negative. It felt like some story you would hear from a World War II survivor. We all received numbers. We became so used to hearing positives that when we heard negatives, it caught our attention. Then we rushed to protect the patient whose number came up negatively.

We worked extra shifts because we had no choice. Days blurred into nights, nights into weeks, and the schedule posted on the wall lost all meaning. You came in even when your body didn't want to move, when your eyes burned from lack of sleep, when you felt hollowed out from grief. There was no such thing as "short-staffed" anymore. There was just *us*, and whoever showed up that day became the team.

The deaths came one after another, so quickly that I stopped counting. The first few hit hard, like punches to the chest. Then came the numbness—a strange, floating kind of exhaustion where you knew you were still functioning, still talking, still moving from bed to bed, but it felt like you were watching yourself from somewhere above. The only thing that kept you grounded was the moments you didn't expect: a coworker handing you a granola bar, someone squeezing your shoulder, eyes locking across a crowded hallway in a silent exchange of *I'm still here. Are you?*

Trauma bonding isn't some poetic metaphor. It's real. We clung to one another because no one else in our lives could understand what we were seeing—bodies bagged one after the other, ventilators maxed out, a patient coding in the next room while you were still charting the death of the one before. We carried each other through shifts with dark jokes and half-smiles, the kind you share not because they're funny, but because they're the only thing preventing you from screaming.

The isolation protocols were brutal. Families weren't allowed in, so they called nonstop, desperate for updates. We became their eyes and ears, their last connection to loved ones they couldn't touch. It was through an iPad—shaking in a nurse's gloved hands—that sons and daughters said goodbye. The conversations were always soft, always broken. "I love you, Dad." "Mom, we're here." "You're not alone." I still hear those words at night sometimes, hovering in the quiet.

And when you walked out of the room afterward, the guilt followed you. We tried to be everything these patients lost: their comfort, their family, their final human touch. But at the end of each shift, it felt like we were leaving pieces of ourselves behind in those rooms—pieces we never got back.

We were doing everything we could, giving everything we had, yet it never felt like enough. That was the worst part. The guilt of survival, the guilt of stepping away from the bedside to grab a sip of water while someone down the hall coded, the guilt of being human in a place that demanded more than humanity could offer.

Every day felt surreal, like walking through a nightmare you couldn't wake from—a dream where everyone around you was fighting invisible flames with empty buckets. You moved fast, but never fast enough. You cared deeply, but never deeply enough. You held yourself together even as everything inside you felt like it was unraveling thread by thread.

We were exhausted beyond words, but we kept going. Because there were still patients who needed us. Because our coworkers needed us. Because stopping wasn't an option—not when the war was still raging around us.

In those months, I learned the true meaning of resilience. Not the kind people about which post on motivational posters, but the raw, unvarnished kind—where you show up broken and terrified, but you show up anyway.

That was our reality. That was our war.

The pandemic introduced new terms like "New Normal," social distancing, flattening the curve, shelter-in-place, and essential workers into everyday language. PPE and nasal passage swabs became commonplace to talk about outside medical settings. Hospitals felt chaotic and tense, with no effective Covid treatment. We felt like we were at war. We knew little about our enemy and had few weapons to take into battle.

AT first—only an improvised mix of vitamins and chloroquine, which often did more harm than good. It was supportive care, oxygen, and symptom management. While public debate raged about the reality of COVID-19, hospital staff were too busy fighting it and caring for patients to argue its existence.

We were beyond capacity almost every day we knew it existed.

Rooms filled faster than they emptied. Stretchers lined the hallways. Spaces that had never held patients before were suddenly converted into care areas. Privacy became a luxury no one could afford. Curtains replaced walls. Monitors were dragged from one room to another, cords stretching across floors like lifelines we hoped wouldn't snap.

There was no room left—not physically, not emotionally.

The alarms never stopped.

They blended together into a constant, disorienting chorus—oxygen levels dropping, heart rates climbing, ventilators struggling to keep up. At some point, the sound stopped registering as individual alerts and became something else entirely. A background noise. A signal that everything, everywhere, was urgent all at once.

We moved faster, but it was never fast enough.

Patients came in gasping for air, their fear immediate and unmistakable. You could see it in their eyes—the realization that something was very wrong, that breathing, something so automatic, had suddenly become work. Heavy, desperate work.

Death came differently now.

It didn't arrive slowly or gently. It came in waves—one after another, sometimes in the same shift, sometimes in the same hour. There was no time to process one loss before the next one began. No time to step away, to breathe, to grieve.

Death after death after death.

At first, each one felt like a shock. Then a blow. Then something harder to define—something duller, heavier. Not because it mattered less, but because there was no space left to feel it fully. The mind adapted in ways the heart couldn't.

Burnout wasn't a future possibility anymore. It was our reality.

You could see it in the way people moved—slower, heavier, like every step required more effort than the last. You could hear it in voices that had lost their edge, flattened by exhaustion. You could feel it in the silence between conversations, where words used to be.

We were running on instinct more than energy.

Tasks became automatic. Muscle memory took over. Assess, medicate, document, repeat. There was comfort in the routine, even as everything around it fell apart. It gave us something to hold onto, something predictable in a world that no longer made sense.

But underneath that routine, the cracks were showing.

Hands trembled slightly when no one was looking. People forgot small things—where they set something down, what they had just been about to say. Names blurred together. Days lost their edges. Everything became one long, continuous stretch of effort.

And still, we kept going.

Because stopping wasn't an option.

There were moments—brief, fragile moments—where the reality of it all broke through. Standing in a room after a patient passed, the machines finally quiet. Looking at the bed, suddenly too still. Realizing there was no family to call in, no one waiting just outside the door.

Just us.

Just witnesses to a life ending in isolation.

Those were the moments that stayed.

Not loud. Not dramatic. Just heavy. Permanent.

The kind that followed you down the hallway, into the break-room, into your car at the end of the shift. The kind that lingered long after you closed your eyes, replaying in fragments you couldn't quite piece together or let go of.

Inside that war zone, time didn't move the same way.

Days stretched. Nights blurred. Weeks disappeared.

All that existed was the next patient, the next alarm, the next breath—if it came.

And somewhere in the middle of it all, we were still there.

Exhausted. Overwhelmed. Still standing.

Still fighting a war, no one could see, except the ones inside it.

Nurses see the best and worst of humanity. Adversity builds character, but it also reveals character. We saw this on a large scale. It was magnified. Outside the hospital, we saw violence, racism, price gouging, and hoarding of supplies, leaving little for others. But we also saw great acts of kindness and courage.

Inside the hospital during intense times, it became more evident. We did what we could to comfort people. We filled gloves with warm water. When we were not there, it could seem like a warm hand was holding theirs. Singing or playing music. Holding rosary beads and praying with them. After all, we were all they had in those moments.

We tried to keep some sense of normalcy in chaos. Talking about what TV shows we watched, food we liked, and reminiscing about our favorite places to go on vacation.

Out of frustration, co-workers lashed out at each other. As nurses became more exhausted, it became more frequent.

As we were balancing caring for our patients and keeping ourselves safe, we were also dealing with the effects of COVID and the shutdown in our personal lives. Many lost family members to Covid and co-workers. The economic impact of their family members losing their jobs made many nurses the sole breadwinners in their homes.

We were humans dealing with the same issues as the rest of the world yet fighting on the frontlines at the same time.

Being a nurse is not just something you do; it is something you are. Caring for people is what we do but trying to balance the outside closure and the inside war zone was difficult at times. No one asked us how we were dealing with or coping. We were given cookies with the word 'HERO' on them. Pizza parties thrown by management. Here is a slice of pizza, a cookie and were told we were heroes.

Outside the hospital, we were also called 'Heroes.' The media would air puff pieces on how some nurse or frontline worker did something kind or heroic. To raise the morale of people and to pat those of us inside the war zone on the back. But in the end, we were just a part of humanity, the best and worst in us. Not superheroes wearing a cape, swooping down to save the day.

Then the heroes became the casualties.

There was a moment when the war stopped being something we were walking into... and became something that turned back on us.

At first, it was just whispers.

"Did you hear? She tested positive."

It would come up quietly, in between tasks, in the hallway, near the medication room. Names spoken carefully, like saying them too loudly, might make it spread faster.

"She was fine last week."
"He just worked three shifts in a row."
"They think it came from a patient."

We kept moving when we heard it. There wasn't time to stop. But something shifted inside each of us, a small crack forming where certainty used to be.

Until then, the virus had been something we were fighting.

Now it was something that was reaching back.

The first time someone we worked closely with got sick, it didn't feel real. They had been right beside of us for days before—laughing, charting, adjusting her mask, doing everything we were told to do. Careful. Capable. Strong.

Then they were gone from the schedule.

At first, it was just "out sick."

Then it became COVID.

We replayed everything.

"Were we close enough?"
"Did we share supplies?"
"Did I touch my face after being near them?"

There was no clear answer. Just a quiet, growing awareness that we were more exposed than we wanted to admit.

More names followed.

One by one.

Then more quickly.

Assignments had to be rearranged mid-shift because someone developed symptoms. Entire groups of staff were suddenly in quarantine. The schedule became something unstable, changing by the hour instead of the week.

We stopped asking *if* it would happen to us.

We started wondering *when*.

The unit felt thinner, even when it was full.

Not just physically, but emotionally. Every absence carried weight. Every empty space at the nurses' station was a reminder that this wasn't just happening to our patients anymore.

It was happening to us.

There was a different kind of fear now.

Before, we feared bringing it home.

Now, we feared already having it.

Every cough meant something. Every headache lingered longer than it should. Fatigue—something we had always known—became suspect.

"Is this just exhaustion... or is it more?"

We checked our temperatures obsessively. Paid attention to every sensation in our bodies. Questioned things we would have ignored before.

But even with that fear, we kept working.

Because there was no alternative.

Patients still needed care. The unit was still full. And every person who got sick meant there were fewer of us left to carry the load.

There were moments when the reality of it all hit harder than others.

Hearing that a coworker had been hospitalized.

Learning that someone was on oxygen.

Waiting for updates that didn't come fast enough.

And the worst ones—the ones we didn't want to think about—when recovery wasn't guaranteed.

We didn't talk about those out loud.

Not fully.

But we felt them.

There was guilt, too.

Guilt for wondering if you had exposed someone.
Guilt for feeling relieved when your test came back negative.
Guilt for still being able to work when someone else couldn't.

It settled into us quietly, another layer added to everything we were already carrying.

And yet, something else happened in those moments.

We took care of each other in ways that didn't need to be spoken.

Covering shifts without hesitation.
Checking in with quick messages: *How are you feeling? Do you need anything?*
Dropping off groceries. Sending food. Offering support in whatever way we could manage.

It wasn't dramatic.

It was steady.

Intentional.

Necessary.

Because if war was coming for us too, then we had to hold the line for each other.

There was no clear separation anymore—no line between caregiver and casualty had become blurred, between nurse and patient. That boundary had blurred, then disappeared altogether.

We were both.

And maybe that was the moment when everything became undeniable.

This wasn't just something we were witnessing.
It wasn't just something we were treating.

We were inside it.

Fully.

And even as it reached into our own ranks, even as it took pieces of our team, our sense of safety, our illusion of control—

We kept showing up.

Because that's what we did.

Even when the war came for us.

What you perceive as the nurse becomes different when you are the patient.

The bed feels different when it's yours.

That's the first thing you notice. As a nurse, a hospital bed is just part of the environment—something you adjust, raise, lower, move around. But lying in it, you realize how small it feels. How exposed. How little control you have once you're in it.

The sounds were the same—but they didn't land the same way.

The beeping of monitors, once just background noise, became something sharper. Personal. Each alarm felt like it belonged to you, even when it didn't. The rhythm of the ICU—the constant hum of machines, ventilators cycling, IV pumps clicking—was no longer something that you worked within.

As a patient, you were now inside of it.

Time changed.

As a nurse, time is structured—med passes, assessments, charting. There's always something next. But as a patient, time stretches. Bends. You wait without knowing for what. Minutes feel longer. Nights feel endless.

You become aware of things you never noticed before.

The weight of the oxygen.
The dryness in your throat.
The way every breath requires just a little more effort than it should.
And the equipment—things nurses handle daily—feel different when they are attached to you.

IV lines are no longer something you started and managed, but something that tethered you in place. Tubing that followed every movement, reminding you that you are not as free as you thought. The pulse ox is gripping your finger, blinking steadily, tracking something you could feel slipping.

As a nurse, you explain these things to patients countless times.

"It might feel uncomfortable."
"Try to relax."
"We're monitoring you closely."
Then you understood what those words didn't fully capture.

The vulnerability.

The loss of control.

The quiet fear that sits just beneath the surface, even when you try to stay calm.

And then there was the proning—carefully positioning pillows, adjusting limbs, explaining the process. It was clinical. Methodical. Necessary.

But being the one turned—face down, supported by pillows, breathing into the mattress—it felt entirely different. It was disorienting. Heavy. A strange mix of relief and discomfort.

You focus on your breathing.

Inhale.
Exhale.
Inhale again.

You become aware of every single breath in a way you never were before.

And somewhere in all of it, your identity shifts.

You're still a nurse. That doesn't disappear.

But in that bed, in that moment—you're also a patient.

And the two don't sit easily together.

You understand too much.

You recognize the sounds, the patterns, the changes in tone when staff speak just outside your room. You know what certain numbers mean. You know what they're watching for.

You know what could happen.

And yet, you're also dependent.

Dependent on the very system you once navigated from the other side.

On the people who now walk into your room the way you used to walk into theirs—focused, efficient, doing their best under impossible circumstances.

There's a strange kind of surrender in that.

Not giving up—but letting go of control in a way that feels unfamiliar, even uncomfortable.

You realize, maybe for the first time, what your patients have been experiencing all along.

Not just physically—but emotionally.

The uncertainty.
The waiting.
The need for reassurance that goes beyond clinical words.

A hand on your arm.
A voice that feels steady.
Someone seeing you—not just your symptoms.

Those things matter more than any monitor can measure.

Lying there, surrounded by the same sounds, the same equipment, the same environment that you thought you knew well.

Not as a workplace.

But as a lifeline.

The ICU wasn't just a place where we fought to save lives.

It was a place where people faced their most vulnerable moments—where control slipped, where fear lived quietly, where hope sometimes came in the smallest forms.

Being in bed as a COVID patient, not standing at the bedside. The line between caregiver and casualty wasn't just blurred. It was gone.

It is scary to lie in a hospital bed with COVID after being the caregiver on the other side. You know the possible outcomes. You think of your family that can't be there for you, and of how they will deal with your death if that is the outcome. You assisted your patients to the bathroom or put them on bedpans, but now you can't breathe well enough to get out of bed. Your colleagues assisted you with a bedpan, providing the same care that you routinely offered to your patients.

Fear came from the uncertainty of the outcome, mixed with dealing with having to rely on your co-workers to help you with basic life functions and not being able to breathe. The same thing that had happened the past few months but now you were on the other side of it.

When people recovered from COVID, the song, 'Here Comes the Sun' by the Beatles was played as the patient was pushed out of the hospital in a wheelchair. It was a celebration. They survived and were going home. Most of the time, they were going home with oxygen, but they were going home. Staff wearing their PPE would gather around the patient as if it were a victory parade. In a sense, it was. As a nurse, to be the patient in the chair wheeled out was a much different experience.

It was a celebration; you survived. You were here to tell the story of how I was the patient. A casualty and a caregiver of COVID. But in the back of your mind, you knew you had to come back and face the enemy even though you had just conquered it.

CHAPTER FIVE

From Heroes to Zeros

"Live your life while you have it. Life is a splendid gift." – Florence Nightingale.

By the summer of 2020, the applause had stopped.

In March and April, people called us heroes. They taped hand-drawn signs to their windows with rainbows and thank-yous. News anchors praised "healthcare warriors," and strangers sent food to the hospital with little notes that said things like *We appreciate you* or *Thank you for saving lives.*

But it didn't take long for the world to lose its patience.

As the months dragged on and the crisis didn't magically disappear, the public's love turned sour. The same people who clapped for us were suddenly calling the virus a hoax. The same people who praised nurses as heroes were shouting at us in the grocery store because we were still wearing masks. The same public that thanked us for risking our lives now accused us of being part of some grand conspiracy to control the population with fear.

It was like whiplash—emotional, violent whiplash.

Everywhere you looked, protests were erupting. Crowds gathering without masks, holding signs that said *COVID IS A LIE, END*

THE SHUTDOWN, NURSES NEED TO STOP SPREADING FEAR. We watched the footage on TV during a break, standing next to a coworker who still had the marks from this N-95 mask etched into her cheeks. We stared at the screen in disbelief and said quietly, "Do they have any idea what we're seeing every day?"

Of course they didn't.

Inside the hospital, people were still dying alone. We were still running out of PPE. We were still exhausted—physically, mentally, spiritually. But outside, people were screaming at governors, storming public buildings, and accusing healthcare workers of inflating death counts for money. It felt like we had stepped into some twisted parallel universe.

For the first time in our careers, it felt like we were hated for doing our jobs.

Some of us were told not to wear scrubs in public because it made us targets. Nurses were yelled at in parking lots. There were stories of healthcare workers being refused service or told they were "part of the problem." Online comment sections were flooded with accusations that hospitals were faking numbers, staging photos, and exaggerating for attention.

Meanwhile, we were holding iPads for dying patients because their families couldn't be there.

That was the part that broke us the most—the disconnect between reality and denial. We had seen things that would never leave us: the blue tint of oxygen-starved lips, the panicked breathing, the weight of another body bag being zipped. We carried the trauma on our skin, in our muscles, in the places of ourselves we tried not to visit too often. And yet, people were standing on street corners yelling that it wasn't real.

The betrayal settled deep.

It wasn't just that the public stopped supporting us. They turned against us. Overnight, it felt like we went from being "heroes" to being disposable, an inconvenience, a reminder of a truth they didn't want to face. We weren't symbols of bravery anymore—we were symbols of a nightmare they were desperate to pretend wasn't happening.

Inside the hospital, we whispered about it in break rooms with tired, stunned voices:

"How can they say it's fake?"
"Do they think our patients are pretending?"
"What else do they want from us?"

There were no answers.

All we knew was that we were still drowning in crisis while the world outside acted like we were making it up. It created a new kind of exhaustion, heavier than the physical kind—the exhaustion of feeling unseen, unvalued, and deeply, painfully alone.

But we kept showing up. Because the patients were still real, even if the disbelief outside tried to erase them. Because we had each other, the only people who truly understood. Because we didn't become nurses for applause—but the cruelty of its absence still stung.

And because, despite everything, it was still our job.

We stayed on the frontlines, even when the world turned its back on us.

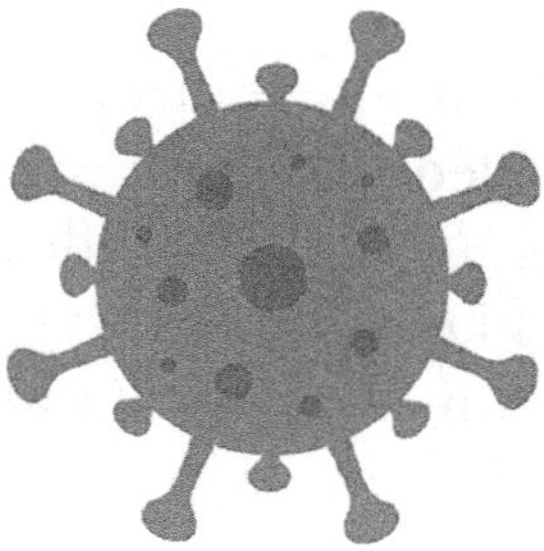

CHAPTER SIX

A Biblical Plague—Wondering if Moses Would Part Some Water or if Jesus Would Walk On some.

"How very little can be done in the spirit of fear." – Florence Nightingale.

By the fall of 2020, it felt like we were walking through the hospital with empty hands. Not because we weren't carrying anything—charts, PPE, medications, iPads, fear—but because emotionally, spiritually, there was nothing left to hold onto. We all felt that way. We were hollowed out versions of ourselves, trying to keep moving forward even as pieces of us kept falling behind.

Colleagues were quitting weekly. Some left quietly, without a goodbye, slipping their badges into HR envelopes and disappearing. Others broke down in the middle of a shift, tears soaking the inside of their masks as they whispered, "I can't do this anymore." We didn't judge them. How could we? Their leaving felt like witnessing someone escaping a burning building while we stayed inside, still searching for survivors. We wished them peace, even as their absence made everything heavier.

Chronic understaffing became the norm. Our patient loads doubled—sometimes tripled. Breaks disappeared. Days off were interrupted by desperate texts begging for help. Every shift felt like entering a storm with no shelter: you just held on and hoped not to get swept away. We were working with bones rather than muscles, with fumes rather than fuel.

And then came the holidays.

We didn't see family on Thanksgiving. Christmas or New Year's. We stayed home, isolating ourselves out of fear of what we might bring with us. Some of us ate dinner alone. Others Face Timed family while sitting in scrubs in dim break rooms, swallowing guilt along with lukewarm meals. Our patients became the only people we saw in person, day after day. Some of them fought bravely and survived. Others didn't.

The grief was constant. Slow. Airless. It wasn't just the patients we lost—it was coworkers, neighbors, our own family members. We attended memorial services over Zoom, a screen became a window into grief that never fully shut. Every death echoed through the unit like a cold draft you couldn't block out.

But there were moments—small, quiet moments—that reminded us of why we stayed.

There were patients who held on with courage that I still don't understand. The ones who looked up at us with exhausted eyes and whispered, "Thank you for not giving up on me." The ones who became familiar faces over weeks or months, who fought their way back to breath, who left the hospital waving a trembling hand as we clapped from the hallway, a bittersweet celebration of survival.

There were acts of kindness that fell like soft snow on a burnt landscape. A coworker leaving a coffee on your workstation with your name written in shaky pen. A stranger donating handmade masks with colorful patterns, bringing a moment of brightness. A patient's family sending cupcakes with a note that said, *You cared for her when we couldn't. Thank you for being her family when we couldn't be there.*

And there were moments between us—the nurses, techs, housekeeping staff, respiratory therapists, doctors—that stitched us together when everything else was unraveling. A shared laugh in the middle of chaos. A knowing glance that said *I see you. I know how hard this is.* A hand on your back after a difficult death. These tiny gestures became our lifelines.

We were carrying grief in both hands, but we were also carrying each other.

That is when we came to a profound realization: healing didn't come from strength, but from connection. From showing up for one another when none of us felt whole. From finding meaning in moments that were small but real.

Carrying on with empty hands didn't mean we had nothing to give. It meant we had given everything—and somehow, we were still finding ways to give a little more.

CHAPTER SEVEN

Here Comes the Sun

"We must accept finite disappointment but never lose infinite hope." – Dr. Martin Luther King Jr.

October going into November felt like we were standing at the edge of a long, dark tunnel and seeing the faintest flicker of light—small, distant, but unmistakably there. After months of death, chaos, isolation, and exhaustion, the arrival of an FDA-approved treatment for COVID felt almost unreal, like something we had dreamed of but never fully believed would happen.

In May, the FDA had given EUA, emergency use authorization, of the drug Remdesivir for COVID. Until then, treatment was about oxygen and symptom management. We felt like we were at war with no weapons against the enemy. The arrival of Remdesivir left us skeptical yet hopeful.

We started by giving a loading dose, then four doses intravenously over five days. At the time, patients were coming into the hospital with mild symptoms, then rapidly declining. Mild symptoms such as shortness of breath with activity, cough, and low-grade fever turned into a code blue within seconds. Due to a sudden drop in oxygen levels, they had to be intubated and put on a breathing machine. We were willing to give it a try to save lives. At first, patients had to give written permission for us to give the medication.

Something unexpected started happening. By the third or fourth dose, patients who could not get out of bed were able to do so and walked to the bathroom without assistance. They needed oxygen and were short of breath with ambulation but could do it on their own.

During the times that patients were lined up in the hallways in gurneys, we were running out of ventilators. More people were not surviving than surviving. The media was showing news clips of refrigerated trucks outside of hospitals being used because the morgues were full.

Because no visitors were allowed inside the hospital, we were making calls to loved ones to say their family members did not make it. The grieving process could not happen as it usually did. People were saying good-bye over video chat and sometimes not at all. They saw their loved one leave the house with mild symptoms to go to the hospital then they never heard from them again nor could they have a memorial service.

We were desperate for answers for a treatment that worked.

We were tired of making calls to family members that started with "I have some bad news."

We finally had a weapon against the enemy.

By October, Remdesivir was approved by the FDA. We had protocols to follow for the treatment of COVID. Outside the hospital the world was beginning to open back up. The illusion of normal.

By October, the world began to open its eyes again.

Not fully. Not all at once. But slowly—carefully, unevenly—like someone testing the weight on an injured leg. Restaurants reopened at limited capacity. Schools debated returning. Airplanes filled with masked passengers. The language shifted from *shutdown* to *reopening*, from *emergency* to *managing the risk*.

On the news, the tone had changed.

There were still reports of rising case numbers, warnings from public health officials, and maps shaded in red and orange. But alongside that came something new—fatigue. A subtle shift in how the pandemic was being talked about. Less urgency. More debate.

"Can we live with the virus?"
"Is it time to reopen the economy?"
"How much longer can restrictions last?"

The conversations weren't just about health anymore. They were about tolerance—what people were willing to accept, what they were willing to ignore.

From inside the hospital, it felt surreal.

Because nothing inside had truly opened back up.

The patients were still coming. Still struggling. Still requiring the same intense level of care. The isolation protocols hadn't gone away. The masks hadn't come off. The fear—quieter now, more internal—was still there.

But outside, it looked different.

Parking lots were fuller. Traffic returned. People gathered again, cautiously at first, then with more confidence. You could feel the world trying to reclaim something it had lost, even if it meant pretending the threat had softened.

It created a strange disconnect.

We would walk out of the hospital after a shift—mentally and physically drained—and step into a world that looked almost normal again. People sitting at outdoor tables, laughing. Stores open. Music playing. Life continuing.

It felt like stepping between two realities.

Inside: controlled, restricted, heavy.
Outside: moving forward, uncertain but determined.

The news didn't ignore the pandemic, but it didn't carry the same urgency either. There were segments about reopening strategies, vaccine progress, and timelines. Words like "*second wave*" and "*surge*" were mentioned, but they didn't land the same way anymore.

Maybe people were tired of hearing it.
Maybe they needed to believe things were getting better.

Inside the hospital, we weren't sure what to believe.

There was a quiet concern among staff—a feeling that this wasn't over, that something was building again beneath the surface. You could hear it in conversations at the nurses' station:

"It feels too soon."
"Cases are still high."
"I think it's going to get bad again."

But those conversations stayed mostly within the walls of the hospital.

Outside, the narrative was shifting toward moving forward.

And maybe that was necessary. People needed hope. They needed movement. They needed something that felt like progress.

But from where we stood, it felt fragile.

Like something being held together by belief more than reality.

October existed in that in-between space—not as heavy as the spring, not as chaotic as the months before, but not safe either. A pause, almost. A breath held collectively, even if not everyone realized they were holding it.

We kept working. Kept watching. Kept waiting.

Because deep down, there was a quiet understanding among us:

The story wasn't finished yet, but it felt like there was light at the end of the tunnel.

Then the vaccine arrived. When the first shipment arrived at the hospital, people gathered to watch as if it was some sacred moment. The box itself wasn't much to look at—plain, cold, clinical—but to many of us, it felt like hope delivered on dry ice. Some nurses cried. Others clapped. Some stared quietly, letting the moment wash over them in a way they couldn't quite express.

But hope didn't come alone. It came tangled with fear, with skepticism, with exhaustion so heavy it muted celebration.

The public's reaction was immediate and divided. Some people were desperate for the vaccine, ready to stand in line for hours. Others swore it was dangerous, rushed, part of a government plot. Social media was a battlefield of conspiracy theories and passionate arguments. In the hospital, we tried to tune it out, but the noise seeped into everything.

Nurses were divided as well. Some took the vaccine right away, some fought not to take it. It became mandatory to receive the

COVID-19 vaccine, many nurses received the vaccine when they were against it just to keep their jobs.

Sitting in a chair, sleeves rolled up, the alcohol pad cold on our skin. When the needle went in, fear in our eyes—not from pain, but from the weight of what this moment meant. For the first time in nearly a year, maybe it was a sliver of protection. A sliver of a future. A mixture of fear and hope.

New medications were emerging, too—treatments that weren't cures, but tools. Monoclonal antibodies. Steroids were refined through trial and error. We started to see patients who would've spiraled months earlier begin to stabilize. We saw oxygen needs decrease, ventilators avoided, and numbers inch upward rather than plummet.

We saw survival.

And with survival came more of the song—*Here Comes the Sun* by The Beatles.

The soft, familiar guitar floated through the speakers, gentle and bright, so painfully out of place against the memory of all we had lost. Staff gathered at the windows as the patient was wheeled out, wrapped in blankets, eyes teary, waving at us with trembling hands. Some of us clapped. Some cried. Some just stood there, letting the warmth of that moment crack open the shell of numbness we had built around ourselves.

"Little darling, the smiles returning to the faces..."

It was impossible not to feel something shift inside us each time that song played. It became a reminder that our work mattered. That survival was possible. That not every story would end in tragedy.

But the vaccine and new treatments didn't fix everything. They didn't erase grief. They didn't bring back the colleagues we lost or undo the trauma we carried. They didn't stop the public arguments, the skepticism, the denial. They didn't lighten the workload overnight. They didn't heal us.

Hope didn't sweep through the halls like a miracle—it seeped in slowly, like sunlight through a crack in a boarded-up window. Warm, but not enough to chase away every shadow.

We were hopeful, yes. But we were conflicted. Worn down. Still grieving. Still bracing.

New Treatments and the vaccine were a turning point, a breath of relief after nearly drowning. But it wasn't the end of the story. It was a beginning—quiet, fragile, and deeply needed.

And for the first time in a long time, as *Here Comes the Sun* played overhead once more, we believed that maybe—just maybe—better days were coming.

CHAPTER EIGHT

THE GOOD, BAD, AND THE UGLY—WHAT 2020 TOOK AND WHAT IT LEFT

"What we see is the remains of the past; to change the future, we must take action in the now with the knowledge we gained." – Martha Hoy

By the end of December 2020, walking the hospital hallways felt like moving through a living scrapbook of the entire year. Every corner, every room, every spot on the linoleum floor held a memory—some we wished we could preserve, many we wished we could forget.

There was a hallway where we lined up beds when we ran out of rooms. I could still see the rows of oxygen tanks humming next to tired bodies fighting for breath. There was the supply room where a coworker had her first panic attack. The break room where we cried together after a coworker died. The door where I had once paused before entering a COVID room, taking one deep breath to steady myself before stepping into the unknown. Even the elevators felt haunted by the year's echoes—muffled sobs, shaky laughter, whispered prayers.

2020 took so much. More than could ever fit neatly onto a calendar.

It took sleep, peace, and the possibility of ever seeing our job the same way again. It took colleagues who should have retired surrounded by family instead of in isolation. It took patients who were more than names on charts—they were people with stories, families, dreams. It took parts of our spirits, pieces of our joy, and for some, even the belief that the world was fundamentally good. It took innocence from a profession that was never that innocent to begin with, but that year stripped away what little we'd been holding onto.

Yet, in a strange way, 2020 gave things too.

It gave us resilience we didn't know we had. It gave us a sense of unity with coworkers who became brothers and sisters in arms. It gave us a clearer understanding of what truly matters—health, family, rest, connection. It gave us moments of tenderness hidden in the chaos, like the time a recovered patient insisted on wheeling themselves out even though they were still weak, tears rolling down their cheeks as *Here Comes the Sun* echoed overhead.

And it gave us each other. That might be the part we treasure the most.

As the year closed, the news was filled with talk of vaccine distribution, debates over mandates, questions about rollout schedules, and cautious optimism from scientists. Some headlines warned of surges and new variants. Others spoke of a "turning point." The world outside was divided, loud, restless—but inside the hospital, the feeling was quieter, more sacred.

Exhaustion still weighed heavily on our bones. Burnout was no longer a threat—it was a shared language. We were tired in a way that didn't go away with sleep, because it was the kind of tired that came from surviving trauma. And yet, despite all of that, something new was present—a thin, flickering thread of hope weaving itself through the halls.

For the first time in months, the ICU wasn't overflowing every single day. For the first time, we had tools that actually made a difference. For the first time, when we admitted a COVID patient, we didn't feel the immediate dread that used to settle heavily on our shoulders. The treatments were imperfect, but better. The vaccine was new, but real. The fear hadn't vanished, but it had softened around the edges.

Hope didn't arrive like a flood—it arrived like dawn. Faint. Slow. Gentle.

When we look back on that year, we were all a different version of ourselves—stronger, more fractured, more human than I ever realized. The world had changed forever. The hallways were lined with ghosts and gratitude in equal measure.

2020 took and gave in the same breath. It broke us, rebuild us, and forced us to confront what it means to care, to sacrifice, to endure. It taught us that hope is not a feeling—it's a choice. One we made over and over, even when our hands were shaking, even when the world wasn't watching.

The hospital felt different—but not healed. The halls were quieter in ways that had nothing to do with patient volume. It was a deeper quiet, the kind that comes after something has passed through and changed everything it touched. We still walked on the same floors, answered the same alarms, cared for the same kinds of patients—but we were not the same people who had stood there at the beginning of the year.

There were moments, standing at the nurses' station or walking past rooms that once held patients whose faces I could still see clearly, when the weight of the year pressed in all at once. It lived in the walls, in the routines, in the silence between conversations. You didn't have to talk about it. Everyone felt it.

2020 took more than we could ever fully name.

It took lives. It took time. It took a sense of safety we once carried without thinking. It took pieces of who we were before we ever understood what we were about to face. There are things from that year that will never leave—the sounds, the images, the moments that replay without warning.

But it also gave something back.

Not in a way that balances the loss, and not in a way I would ever wish for—but it gave clarity. It stripped away what didn't matter and left behind what did. It showed us the depth of human connection, even through layers of isolation. It showed us what it means to keep showing up when there is nothing left to give.

It showed us each other.

As the year closed, there was still exhaustion in every step, still grief that hadn't found a place to settle. But there was also something else—quiet, steady, and real.

Hope.

Not loud. Not certain. But present.

It lived in the patients who walked out of the hospital after weeks of fighting. In the small advances in treatment. In the first vaccines being given. In the simple fact that we had made it through something we once thought we couldn't.

Hope didn't erase what happened. It didn't fix what was broken.

But it made space for what could come next.

And maybe that's what the end of 2020 really was—not a conclusion, not a clean ending, but a threshold. A moment between what we had survived and what we were still becoming.

We walked out of that year changed. Carrying more than we ever expected. Letting go of what we could, holding onto what mattered.

And somewhere, just beyond the exhaustion, just beyond the grief—the sun was beginning to rise again.

Made in the USA
Monee, IL
04 November 2026

67380035R00039